Peaches and Cream: A guide to Dermatological Health Care

Chapter 1: Introduction to Skin Health and Nutrition

The Importance of Skin Health

The health of the skin is a critical aspect of overall well-being and warrants special attention from both health professionals and individuals. As the body's largest organ, the skin serves vital functions, including protection against environmental hazards, regulation of body temperature, and sensation. Maintaining skin health is essential not only for aesthetic reasons but also for preventing various dermatological conditions that can significantly impact quality of life. Understanding the multifaceted nature of skin health is crucial for health professionals who guide patients in their skincare practices and for adults invested in their well-being.

Natural remedies have gained popularity as individuals seek holistic treatments for various skin conditions. This growing interest highlights the importance of understanding herbal solutions and their efficacy in addressing issues such as eczema, psoriasis, and acne. Health professionals should be well-versed in these alternatives to provide informed recommendations that align with each patient's preferences and needs. Additionally, integrating natural remedies with conventional treatments can enhance therapeutic outcomes and promote a more comprehensive approach to skin health.

Tattoo aftercare is another significant aspect of skin health that deserves attention, particularly given the increasing prevalence of body art. Proper aftercare is essential for maintaining skin integrity and preventing complications such as infections or allergic reactions. Health professionals should educate clients on the importance of using appropriate products, including barrier creams and moisturizers, to support healing. This knowledge is vital not only for the immediate post-tattoo period but also for fostering long-term skin health, as tattoos can impact skin texture and hydration if not cared for properly.

Understanding skin types across cultures adds further depth to the conversation about skin health. Different races and ethnicities often have unique skin characteristics that influence their susceptibility to various conditions and the effectiveness of certain treatments. Health professionals must consider these cultural differences when advising on skincare routines and products, fostering inclusivity and respect for diverse beauty practices. This understanding can help bridge gaps in dermatological care and promote healthier skin outcomes across populations.

Nutrition plays a pivotal role in skin health; thus, it is essential to investigate how dietary choices influence skin conditions and aging. A balanced diet rich in vitamins, minerals, and antioxidants can enhance skin resilience and appearance, while deficiencies can exacerbate existing problems. Health professionals should emphasize the importance of nutrition in their discussions with patients, advocating for dietary adjustments that support skin health.

Additionally, raising awareness about skin cancer and the significance of protective measures against UV exposure is crucial in promoting long-term skin health. By integrating these elements into patient education, professionals can empower individuals to take proactive steps in maintaining their skin health and preventing potential issues.

Overview of Diet and Dermatological Health

The relationship between diet and dermatological health is increasingly recognized within the fields of nutrition and dermatology. Health professionals are beginning to understand that the skin, often referred to as the body's largest organ, reflects the overall health of an individual, including dietary choices. A well-balanced diet rich in vitamins, minerals, and essential fatty acids can promote skin vitality and resilience, while poor dietary habits may contribute to various skin conditions such as acne, eczema, and psoriasis. This subchapter will explore how nutrition plays a pivotal role in maintaining skin integrity and addressing specific dermatological concerns.

Research has demonstrated that certain nutrients are particularly beneficial for skin health. For instance, antioxidants such as vitamins C and E help combat oxidative stress, which can lead to premature skin aging and the development of skin disorders. Omega-3 fatty acids, found in fish and flaxseeds, are known to reduce inflammation, making them an important dietary consideration for individuals suffering from conditions like eczema and psoriasis. Additionally, a diet rich in hydration—primarily from fruits and vegetables—supports the skin's moisture barrier, enhancing its overall appearance and function. Health professionals should consider these dietary components when advising patients on skin care practices.

In the realm of holistic treatments and natural remedies, food choices can also directly influence skin conditions. Traditional practices in various cultures often emphasize the connection between dietary habits and skin health. For example, the Mediterranean diet, abundant in olive oil, nuts, and fish, has been associated with reduced skin inflammation and improved hydration. This subchapter will also touch upon how herbal solutions, such as the inclusion of turmeric and green tea, can provide additional anti-inflammatory and antioxidant benefits, further supporting skin health.

The importance of nutrition extends beyond merely treating existing conditions; it also plays a crucial role in skin cancer awareness and prevention. Diets high in fruits and vegetables, particularly those rich in carotenoids and flavonoids, have been linked to a lower risk of developing certain types of skin cancer. On the other hand, excessive consumption of processed foods and sugars can lead to insulin spikes and inflammatory responses, which may exacerbate skin issues and increase vulnerability to skin cancers. Educating patients about the long-term benefits of a nutritious diet can serve as a proactive measure in skin cancer prevention.

Finally, understanding skin types across cultures provides valuable insights into how diverse dietary practices influence dermatological health. Different ethnic groups may have unique dietary staples that contribute to their skin health, revealing a rich tapestry of beauty practices informed by nutritional choices. In addition to cultural considerations, this subchapter will address the implications of diet in tattoo aftercare, highlighting how certain foods can aid in the healing process and promote skin integrity post-tattooing. By integrating these perspectives, health professionals can adopt a more comprehensive approach to dermatological health that encompasses both dietary guidance and holistic treatment modalities.

Chapter 2: The Role of Nutrition in Skin Health

Essential Nutrients for Healthy Skin

Essential nutrients are fundamental to maintaining healthy skin, as they play a pivotal role in its structure, function, and overall appearance. Among these nutrients, vitamins, minerals, fatty acids, and antioxidants contribute significantly to skin health, influencing everything from hydration to the skin's ability to repair itself. Health professionals must understand the specific roles these nutrients play in dermatological care, especially when advising patients on holistic treatments and dietary practices that promote skin integrity.

Vitamins A, C, and E are particularly important for skin health. Vitamin A is crucial for cell turnover, helping to prevent the buildup of dead skin cells that can lead to clogged pores and acne. It also aids in the healing process post-tattoo, making it essential for aftercare. Vitamin C, known for its antioxidant properties, protects the skin from free radical damage while also contributing to collagen synthesis, which is vital for maintaining skin elasticity and reducing signs of aging. Vitamin E complements this by providing additional antioxidant support and enhancing the skin's barrier function, making it particularly beneficial for individuals managing conditions like incontinence, where skin integrity is critical.

Minerals such as zinc and selenium also play essential roles in skin health. Zinc is known for its anti-inflammatory properties and is vital for wound healing, which is particularly important for those dealing with skin injuries or post-tattoo care. Selenium, on the other hand, protects the skin from UV damage and supports the immune system, which can be beneficial in skin cancer awareness and prevention strategies. Incorporating foods rich in these minerals into one's diet can significantly enhance the skin's resilience and healing capabilities.

Fatty acids, particularly omega-3 and omega-6, are essential for maintaining the skin's lipid barrier. These fatty acids help to regulate moisture retention, reducing dryness and irritation. For individuals exploring natural remedies for skin conditions, incorporating sources of these fatty acids, such as flaxseeds, walnuts, and fatty fish, can lead to noticeable improvements in skin texture and hydration. Additionally, understanding the balance of these fatty acids in the diet can aid in managing various skin issues across different cultures, reflecting the diverse beauty practices that exist globally.

Lastly, antioxidants found in fruits, vegetables, and herbal solutions are crucial in combating oxidative stress, which accelerates skin aging and can exacerbate skin conditions. A diet rich in colorful produce not only nourishes the skin but also supports overall health, making it a vital aspect of a holistic approach to dermatological care. As health professionals, recognizing the synergy between nutrition and skin health will empower individuals to make informed dietary choices that promote skin vitality and mitigate various skin challenges.

The Impact of Dietary Choices on Skin Conditions

Dietary choices play a pivotal role in influencing skin health, with emerging research highlighting the intricate connection between nutrition and dermatological conditions. The skin, being the body's largest organ, reflects internal health and vitality. Nutrient deficiencies, excesses, and imbalances can manifest as various skin issues, ranging from acne and eczema to premature aging. Health professionals must recognize that dietary modifications can serve as both preventative and therapeutic measures for patients suffering from skin ailments. By understanding the significance of nutrition, practitioners can offer holistic strategies that complement traditional dermatological treatments.

A diet rich in antioxidants, vitamins, and essential fatty acids is crucial for maintaining skin integrity and combating skin disorders. Antioxidants, found abundantly in fruits and vegetables, help neutralize free radicals that can lead to oxidative stress and skin damage. Vitamins A, C, and E are particularly beneficial for skin repair and rejuvenation. For instance, vitamin C is essential for collagen synthesis, while vitamin A aids in cellular turnover, making them indispensable for treating conditions like acne and photoaging. Similarly, omega-3 fatty acids, commonly found in fatty fish and flaxseeds, have anti-inflammatory properties that can alleviate symptoms of conditions such as psoriasis and dermatitis.

Conversely, certain dietary components can exacerbate skin issues. High glycemic index foods, refined sugars, and dairy products have been linked to increased acne flare-ups and inflammatory responses in susceptible individuals. These foods can spike insulin levels, leading to an overproduction of sebum and clogged pores. Health professionals should educate patients about the potential impact of these dietary choices on their skin, encouraging a balanced diet that prioritizes whole foods over processed options. Such dietary guidance can empower patients to take an active role in their skin health.

Additionally, the cultural context of dietary habits must be considered when addressing skin health across diverse populations. Different cultures have unique beauty practices and dietary preferences that influence skin conditions and their management. For example, traditional diets rich in fermented foods have been associated with improved gut health and, consequently, better skin outcomes. By exploring these cultural variances, health professionals can tailor dietary recommendations that resonate with their patients' backgrounds, enhancing adherence and overall effectiveness.

In conclusion, the impact of dietary choices on skin conditions is profound and multifaceted. By integrating nutritional counseling into dermatological practice, health professionals can significantly improve patient outcomes. Recognizing the relationship between diet and skin health allows for a comprehensive approach to treatment that not only addresses existing conditions but also promotes long-term skin wellness. As research continues to unfold in this area, practitioners should stay informed about the latest findings to offer evidence-based dietary advice that supports both skin health and overall well-being.

Foods That Promote Radiant Skin

Foods that promote radiant skin play a crucial role in achieving and maintaining optimal dermatological health. Nutrition is a cornerstone of skin vitality, influencing everything from hydration levels to the skin's ability to repair itself. A well-balanced diet rich in vitamins, minerals, antioxidants, and healthy fats can mitigate the effects of aging, prevent skin conditions, and enhance overall appearance. For health professionals and adults seeking to improve skin health through dietary choices, understanding the specific foods that contribute to a radiant complexion is essential.

Fruits and vegetables are among the most powerful allies in promoting skin health. Foods such as berries, oranges, and leafy greens are packed with vitamins C and E, which are known for their antioxidant properties. These nutrients help combat oxidative stress caused by environmental factors, such as UV exposure and pollution, which can lead to premature aging and skin damage. Additionally, the high water content in many fruits and vegetables aids in hydration, supporting skin elasticity and overall appearance. Encouraging patients and clients to incorporate a variety of colorful produce into their diets can effectively enhance their skin's radiance.

Healthy fats, particularly omega-3 fatty acids, also play a significant role in skin health. Found in fatty fish like salmon, walnuts, and flaxseeds, omega-3s help maintain the skin's lipid barrier, which is crucial for retaining moisture and preventing dryness. This is particularly relevant for individuals with conditions such as eczema or psoriasis, where maintaining skin hydration is vital. Moreover, these healthy fats possess anti-inflammatory properties, which can alleviate redness and irritation, further contributing to a more radiant complexion. Health professionals should emphasize the importance of including sources of omega-3s in dietary recommendations for skin health.

Moreover, the incorporation of certain nuts and seeds can significantly benefit skin appearance. Almonds, for example, are rich in vitamin E, which aids in protecting the skin from UV damage and supports healing processes. Similarly, sunflower seeds contain selenium, a mineral that plays a role in skin elasticity and protection against environmental stressors. Educating patients about the benefits of these nutrient-dense foods can empower them to make informed dietary choices that support their dermatological health goals.

Finally, hydration cannot be overlooked as a vital component of skin health. While water is essential, foods with high water content, such as cucumbers, tomatoes, and watermelons, can contribute to overall hydration levels. Inadequate hydration can lead to dry, dull skin and exacerbate various skin conditions. Health professionals should advocate for a holistic approach to skincare that includes sufficient fluid intake and the consumption of hydrating foods, underscoring the interconnectedness of nutrition and skin health. By promoting an understanding of these dietary elements, adults can take proactive steps toward achieving and maintaining a radiant complexion.

Chapter 3: Natural Remedies for Skin Conditions

Holistic Treatments for Common Skin Issues

Holistic treatments for common skin issues represent a growing interest among health professionals and adults seeking alternative solutions to conventional dermatological care. These approaches emphasize the interconnectedness of the body, mind, and environment, advocating for a comprehensive understanding of skin health. By exploring natural remedies, herbal solutions, and lifestyle modifications, practitioners can provide patients with effective strategies to manage various skin conditions. This subchapter delves into the principles of holistic treatments while addressing specific skin concerns, including the role of nutrition, cultural practices, and post-tattoo care.

Nutrition plays a crucial role in maintaining skin health and preventing common dermatological issues. A diet rich in antioxidants, vitamins, and essential fatty acids can significantly impact skin conditions such as acne, eczema, and psoriasis. For instance, incorporating foods high in omega-3 fatty acids, like fatty fish and flaxseeds, can help reduce inflammation and promote skin barrier function. Additionally, a focus on hydration and the consumption of fruits and vegetables rich in vitamins C and E can enhance skin elasticity and overall appearance. Health professionals should guide patients in adopting dietary changes that align with their skin health goals, emphasizing the importance of whole foods and limiting processed items.

Cultural perspectives on skin health also provide valuable insights into holistic treatments. Different cultures have distinct beauty practices that reflect their understanding of skin care. For example, traditional Chinese medicine often utilizes herbal remedies and acupuncture to address skin issues from an internal perspective, while Indigenous practices may emphasize the use of natural plants and oils for topical application. By studying these diverse approaches, health professionals can offer more inclusive and culturally sensitive care. Understanding how various races and ethnic groups approach skin health can enhance treatment strategies, ensuring they resonate with patients' backgrounds and beliefs.

Tattoo aftercare exemplifies the importance of maintaining skin integrity and health post-procedure. Holistic treatments in this context often include the application of natural emollients, such as coconut oil or shea butter, to promote healing and minimize irritation. Additionally, educating individuals about the importance of hydration and a balanced diet can further support their skin during the healing process. Health professionals should stress the significance of avoiding harsh chemicals and fragrances in post-tattoo care, opting instead for gentle, natural products that align with holistic principles. This approach not only aids in the healing of the tattooed area but also contributes to the overall health of the skin.

In conclusion, holistic treatments for common skin issues offer a multifaceted approach to dermatological care. By integrating natural remedies, understanding cultural practices, and emphasizing the role of nutrition, health professionals can provide comprehensive support to patients facing various skin concerns. As the demand for alternative solutions grows, it is essential to remain informed about effective holistic practices that promote skin health while respecting individual needs and preferences. Through a combination of education, personalized care, and a commitment to natural healing, practitioners can empower patients to achieve healthier skin and a greater sense of well-being.

Herbal Solutions and Their Efficacy

Herbal solutions have gained increased attention in recent years as a viable option for addressing various dermatological conditions, prompting a shift in how health professionals and adults approach skin health. These natural remedies, derived from plants and herbs, offer a range of therapeutic properties that can complement conventional treatments. The efficacy of herbal solutions, however, can vary widely depending on the specific ingredients, the conditions being treated, and individual skin types. This subchapter aims to explore the potential benefits and limitations of herbal treatments, providing a comprehensive overview for those seeking to incorporate these remedies into their skincare practices.

One of the most promising aspects of herbal solutions is their multi-faceted approach to addressing skin issues. For example, chamomile and calendula have long been recognized for their anti-inflammatory and soothing properties, making them effective in treating conditions such as eczema and dermatitis. Similarly, aloe vera is well-documented for its moisturizing and healing capabilities, particularly in the context of post-tattoo care, where maintaining skin integrity is crucial. Understanding the specific phytochemicals present in these herbs can help health professionals recommend appropriate formulations tailored to individual needs, enhancing therapeutic outcomes.

Despite their potential benefits, it is essential to remain cautious regarding the efficacy of herbal solutions. The scientific evidence supporting many herbal treatments is still in its infancy, with varying results from clinical studies. Factors such as preparation methods, dosage, and individual skin responses can significantly influence outcomes. Thus, health professionals must critically evaluate the available research and consider integrating herbal remedies with established dermatological treatments. This holistic approach not only respects the complexities of skin conditions but also empowers patients to make informed choices about their skincare regimens.

In addition to addressing specific skin conditions, herbal solutions can also play a role in the broader context of skin health and nutrition. Many herbs are rich in antioxidants, vitamins, and minerals that support overall skin integrity and combat the signs of aging. For instance, ingredients like green tea and turmeric offer protective benefits against environmental stressors and inflammation. By understanding the nutritional components of these herbs, health professionals can provide valuable guidance on how dietary choices can influence skin health, further enhancing the effectiveness of topical treatments.

Finally, it is crucial to consider the cultural dimensions of herbal solutions in skincare. Traditional practices across different cultures often utilize local herbs and plants, reflecting a deep understanding of their healing properties. By incorporating these diverse perspectives, health professionals can enrich their practices and better address the unique skin health needs of various populations. Ultimately, the integration of herbal solutions into dermatological healthcare requires a balanced approach that respects traditional knowledge while aligning with contemporary scientific understanding, ensuring that patients receive comprehensive care tailored to their individual skin health journeys.

Integrating Natural Remedies into Daily Skincare

Integrating natural remedies into daily skincare routines represents a paradigm shift in dermatological health care, merging traditional practices with modern scientific understanding. For health professionals and adults alike, this integration offers a holistic approach to addressing various skin conditions while promoting overall skin health. Natural remedies, often derived from plants and herbs, can complement conventional treatments and provide additional benefits, such as reducing inflammation, enhancing hydration, and improving skin elasticity. By understanding the properties of these remedies, practitioners can better guide their patients and clients in creating customized skincare regimens that align with their individual needs.

The diversity of skin types across cultures necessitates a tailored approach to skincare that respects individual differences and preferences. Many traditional cultures have long relied on natural ingredients for skin care, often using locally sourced plants and herbs with proven efficacy. For instance, aloe vera, revered in various cultures, is known for its soothing and healing properties, making it an excellent choice for treating sunburn or irritation. Similarly, turmeric, celebrated for its anti-inflammatory and antioxidant benefits, can be incorporated into skincare routines to combat conditions such as acne or eczema. By examining these cultural practices, health professionals can enrich their understanding of natural remedies, helping to foster a more inclusive perspective on skincare that acknowledges the wisdom of diverse traditions.

Nutrition plays a pivotal role in skin health, further emphasizing the importance of integrating dietary considerations into skincare regimens. Specific nutrients, such as vitamins A, C, and E, along with essential fatty acids, can profoundly impact skin condition and appearance. Natural remedies, including herbal supplements and nutrient-rich foods, can enhance these benefits. For example, incorporating foods high in omega-3 fatty acids, such as flaxseeds and walnuts, can improve skin hydration and elasticity. Moreover, the synergistic effect of combining nutritional insights with topical natural remedies creates a comprehensive approach to skin health, allowing individuals to address underlying issues while also promoting surface-level improvements.

Awareness of skin cancer and its prevention is paramount when considering natural remedies in skincare. While natural ingredients can provide protective benefits, such as antioxidants that combat free radicals, they are not substitutes for sun protection. Health professionals should emphasize the importance of integrating natural remedies with established protective measures, such as broad-spectrum sunscreen use. Ingredients like green tea extract and raspberry seed oil have shown promise in providing additional defense against UV damage, and incorporating them into daily routines can enhance skin protection. This dual approach reinforces the necessity of vigilance in skin care while exploring the beneficial aspects of natural remedies.

Lastly, the management of skin issues related to incontinence and allergic reactions presents unique challenges that can be addressed through natural remedies. Barrier creams infused with natural ingredients, such as shea butter and zinc oxide, provide effective protection against moisture-related skin damage, while herbal solutions like calendula can soothe irritation and promote healing. Education on the proper selection and application of these remedies can empower individuals to maintain skin integrity and prevent complications. By integrating natural remedies into daily skincare practices, health professionals can support their patients in achieving healthier skin while fostering a greater understanding of holistic approaches to dermatological health care.

Chapter 4: Tattoo Aftercare and Skin Health

Best Practices for Tattoo Aftercare

Tattoo aftercare is a crucial aspect of ensuring the longevity and vibrancy of the artwork while maintaining skin health. Following a tattoo procedure, the skin undergoes an intricate healing process that requires careful attention. This subchapter outlines best practices for tattoo aftercare, emphasizing the importance of cleanliness, hydration, and protection. Health professionals and adults alike must understand that proper aftercare not only enhances the appearance of the tattoo but also minimizes the risk of infections and other complications that could arise during the healing phase.

Initially, maintaining a sterile environment is paramount. After getting a tattoo, the area should be gently cleansed with mild, fragrance-free soap and lukewarm water. It is advisable to avoid scrubbing the tattooed area, as this can disrupt the healing skin and lead to irritation. Once cleaned, the area should be pat-dried with a clean towel to prevent moisture accumulation, which can create an environment conducive to bacterial growth. Health professionals can recommend specific cleansers that are formulated for sensitive skin, thereby ensuring that patients are well-informed about the best products to use during this crucial stage.

Hydration plays a vital role in the healing process of a tattoo. Applying a thin layer of a fragrance-free, non-comedogenic moisturizer can help retain moisture and promote healing.

Natural remedies, such as aloe vera and coconut oil, are often suggested for their soothing properties; however, it is essential to ensure that these products do not contain added fragrances or irritants. Health professionals should guide patients in selecting appropriate products, emphasizing the need to avoid petroleum-based ointments, which can suffocate the skin and hinder the natural healing process.

Protection from external irritants is another critical component of tattoo aftercare. It is advisable for individuals to avoid direct sunlight, swimming pools, and hot tubs during the initial healing period, which typically lasts for two to four weeks. The ultraviolet rays from the sun can damage the healing skin and fade the tattoo's colors. For those with a history of skin conditions or sensitivities, discussing the use of barrier creams may be beneficial, as these can provide an additional layer of protection against environmental factors. Health professionals should educate patients about the significance of wearing loose-fitting clothing over the tattooed area to minimize friction and irritation.

Lastly, monitoring the healing process is essential. Patients should be aware of signs of infection, such as increased redness, swelling, or discharge, and seek medical attention if these symptoms arise. Regular follow-up appointments with health professionals can ensure that the healing process is progressing smoothly. By adhering to these best practices for tattoo aftercare, individuals can enjoy their body art while promoting skin health and preventing complications, ultimately leading to a fulfilling and aesthetically pleasing outcome.

Nutrition's Role in Healing Tattooed Skin

Nutrition plays a pivotal role in the healing process of tattooed skin, influencing both immediate recovery and long-term skin health. After undergoing the tattooing process, the skin experiences a form of trauma, which requires proper care and nourishment to facilitate healing. Nutrients such as vitamins, minerals, and antioxidants are essential for promoting skin regeneration, reducing inflammation, and preventing complications like infections or excessive scarring. Understanding how specific dietary choices impact skin recovery can empower health professionals to provide comprehensive aftercare advice to clients, ensuring they maintain the integrity and appearance of their tattoos.

Vitamins A, C, and E, along with essential fatty acids, are particularly beneficial for skin healing. Vitamin A is crucial for cell regeneration and repair, aiding in the turnover of skin cells that may be damaged during the tattooing process. Vitamin C, an antioxidant, not only helps in collagen synthesis but also protects the skin from oxidative stress that can occur post-tattooing. Vitamin E contributes to skin hydration and supports the skin barrier, which is vital for preventing infections. Furthermore, incorporating omega-3 and omega-6 fatty acids into the diet can enhance the skin's lipid barrier, facilitating moisture retention and reducing inflammation, thus promoting a smoother healing process.

Hydration is another critical aspect of nutrition that significantly affects tattooed skin. Adequate water intake is essential for maintaining skin elasticity and overall health.

Dehydrated skin can lead to complications such as prolonged healing, increased itchiness, and a greater likelihood of scabbing or peeling, which can negatively impact the appearance of the tattoo. Health professionals should encourage patients to prioritize hydration, not only through water consumption but also by including hydrating foods such as fruits and vegetables in their diet. This holistic approach to nutrition can optimize both the healing process and the longevity of the tattoo.

In addition to focusing on specific nutrients, a balanced diet rich in whole foods can enhance the body's ability to heal. Whole grains, lean proteins, and a variety of colorful fruits and vegetables provide essential nutrients that support the immune system, reduce inflammation, and promote overall skin health. Furthermore, avoiding processed foods high in sugar and unhealthy fats can prevent exacerbation of skin conditions and ensure that the tattooed area receives the best possible care. Health professionals should advocate for dietary choices that not only aid in recovery but also contribute to long-term skin health, fostering a comprehensive understanding of the relationship between nutrition and dermatological outcomes.

Lastly, educating clients about the potential impact of food sensitivities and allergies on skin healing is crucial. Certain individuals may experience adverse reactions to specific foods, leading to inflammation or delayed healing. Understanding one's unique skin type and dietary tolerances can significantly affect the healing process of tattooed skin. By integrating nutritional education into tattoo aftercare protocols, health professionals can empower clients to make informed choices that promote optimal healing and maintain the beauty of their tattoos. This proactive approach not only enhances the immediate recovery experience but also supports long-term skin health, fostering a deeper appreciation for the intricate relationship between nutrition and dermatological care.

Long-term Care for Tattooed Skin

Long-term care for tattooed skin is an essential aspect of dermatological health that requires attention from both health professionals and individuals with tattoos. The process of tattooing involves introducing ink into the dermis, which can influence skin integrity and health over time. Proper care not only ensures the longevity of the tattoo but also helps prevent various skin conditions that can arise from neglecting the unique needs of tattooed skin. This subchapter will explore effective strategies for maintaining the quality of tattooed skin, focusing on holistic approaches, nutrition, and protective measures.

First and foremost, understanding the specific needs of tattooed skin is crucial for long-term care. The healing process following a tattoo can vary significantly based on skin type, individual health, and aftercare practices. It is important for health professionals to educate clients about the significance of moisturizing and protecting the skin during the healing phase, as this can prevent complications such as infections, scarring, and color fading. Natural remedies, including herbal solutions like aloe vera and calendula, can provide soothing and anti-inflammatory benefits, promoting healthier skin recovery. Furthermore, recommending barrier creams can offer an additional layer of protection, especially for individuals prone to skin sensitivities or allergy reactions.

Nutrition plays a vital role in the maintenance of skin health, particularly for those with tattoos. A diet rich in antioxidants, vitamins, and minerals can enhance skin repair and resilience. Health professionals should encourage their clients to consume foods high in omega-3 fatty acids, such as salmon and walnuts, which can help maintain skin elasticity and hydration. Additionally, hydration is key; drinking ample water supports skin health from within, ensuring that the skin remains supple and vibrant. A holistic approach to nutrition not only contributes to the appearance of the tattoo but also aids in overall skin health, reducing the risk of conditions like dermatitis or eczema that could arise post-tattooing.

In the context of skin cancer awareness, tattooed individuals must remain vigilant about skin health. Tattoos may obscure changes in the skin, making routine examinations by dermatologists essential for early detection of potential skin issues, including cancer. Health professionals should stress the importance of regular skin checks and educate clients about the signs of skin cancer, such as unusual moles or changes in existing tattoos. Additionally, the use of sunscreen on tattooed areas should be a non-negotiable practice, as UV exposure can lead to fading and increase the risk of skin damage. Recommendations for broad-spectrum, water-resistant sunscreens can protect the skin while preserving the integrity of the tattoo.

Finally, addressing skin conditions associated with incontinence is critical in the long-term care of tattooed skin, particularly for individuals susceptible to skin damage. The application of barrier creams can prevent skin breakdown and irritation, particularly in areas where tattoos exist. It is also essential for health professionals to advocate for proper hygiene practices and the use of moisture-wicking materials to minimize the risk of infections. By incorporating first aid techniques for common skin injuries, practitioners can empower clients with knowledge on how to manage potential skin issues effectively. This comprehensive approach ensures that individuals with tattoos can enjoy their body art while maintaining optimal skin health throughout their lives.

Chapter 5: Understanding Skin Types Across Cultures

Cultural Perspectives on Skin Health

Cultural perspectives on skin health reflect a complex interplay of traditions, beliefs, and practices that vary significantly across different societies. These perspectives shape how individuals perceive skin conditions, treatments, and overall skin health, influencing both personal care routines and professional dermatological practices. In many cultures, skin is not just a physical barrier but a canvas that conveys identity, beauty, and even social status. Understanding these cultural nuances is essential for health professionals who aim to provide inclusive and effective care tailored to diverse populations.

Natural remedies for skin conditions are often rooted in cultural traditions and herbal knowledge passed down through generations. For instance, in some indigenous cultures, specific plants and herbs are revered for their healing properties, employed not only in the treatment of skin ailments but also as preventive measures. These practices highlight a holistic approach, where skin health is viewed in conjunction with overall well-being. Health professionals should consider integrating these natural remedies into their treatment plans, particularly for patients who may prefer or respond better to non-pharmaceutical interventions.

Tattoo aftercare is another area where cultural practices significantly influence skin health. In societies where tattooing is a rite of passage or a form of self-expression, the methods used for aftercare can vary widely. Some cultures may emphasize the use of specific oils or balms derived from local flora to promote healing, while others might advocate for minimal intervention to allow the skin to recover naturally. Understanding these cultural approaches can enhance the effectiveness of aftercare recommendations and improve patient compliance, as individuals often feel more connected to practices that resonate with their cultural backgrounds.

The role of nutrition in skin health is universally acknowledged, yet dietary practices differ across cultures. Traditional diets rich in antioxidants, vitamins, and healthy fats can significantly impact skin conditions, aging, and overall beauty. For example, Mediterranean diets, which emphasize olive oil and fresh produce, are often associated with healthier skin, while high-sugar or processed food diets may correlate with increased skin issues such as acne. Health professionals should promote culturally relevant nutritional advice, recognizing that dietary changes may be more readily embraced when they align with existing cultural practices and preferences.

Lastly, skin cancer awareness and prevention efforts must be culturally sensitive to be effective. Risk factors and perceptions of skin cancer can vary widely across different ethnic groups. For example, individuals with darker skin may underestimate their risk due to common misconceptions about skin cancer prevalence. Tailoring educational materials and outreach programs to reflect cultural beliefs and practices can enhance awareness and encourage proactive skin health behaviors. By fostering open dialogues about skin health that respect and incorporate cultural perspectives, health professionals can improve outcomes and promote a more inclusive approach to dermatological care.

Traditional Beauty Practices and Their Nutritional Basis

Traditional beauty practices have long been intertwined with nutritional wisdom, offering insights into how ancient cultures utilized readily available ingredients to promote skin health. These practices often highlight the connection between the food we consume and the condition of our skin, emphasizing the importance of a holistic approach to beauty. By examining these time-honored rituals, health professionals can gain a deeper understanding of how nutrition influences dermatological health and can incorporate these insights into modern treatment plans.

Many traditional beauty practices utilize natural ingredients that are rich in vitamins, antioxidants, and essential fatty acids. For instance, the application of honey, a staple in many cultures, not only serves as a humectant but also possesses antimicrobial properties that can benefit the skin. Similarly, the use of olive oil in Mediterranean cultures is renowned for its moisturizing and anti-inflammatory effects, which can support skin health, especially in individuals with dry or aging skin. These examples illustrate how nutritional components can enhance dermatological care, reinforcing the idea that what we apply topically should be complemented by what we consume.

The cultural significance of these practices also varies widely, reflecting diverse understandings of skin health across different races and societies. In some Asian cultures, for example, the consumption of green tea is believed to provide protection against skin damage due to its high levels of polyphenols, which can help mitigate oxidative stress. Meanwhile, Indigenous practices often emphasize the use of local herbs and foods, such as aloe vera and coconut oil, which are recognized for their soothing and healing properties. By exploring these varied approaches, health professionals can appreciate the unique nutritional foundations that underpin skin care across cultures.

The role of nutrition in skin health is further underscored by contemporary research linking dietary choices to common skin conditions. For instance, diets rich in omega-3 fatty acids, found in fish and nuts, have been shown to reduce inflammation, potentially alleviating symptoms associated with conditions like eczema and psoriasis. Additionally, the impact of sugar and processed foods on skin aging and elasticity has gained attention, prompting a re-evaluation of dietary habits in the context of maintaining youthful skin. These findings emphasize the necessity of integrating nutritional counseling into dermatological practice, allowing for a more comprehensive approach to skin health.

Finally, as we recognize the significance of traditional beauty practices and their nutritional basis, it becomes essential to educate patients on the importance of both diet and lifestyle in their skin care routines. Health professionals should advocate for a balanced diet that includes a variety of fruits, vegetables, whole grains, and healthy fats, while also encouraging the exploration of traditional remedies that align with modern scientific understanding. By fostering this holistic approach, we can empower individuals to take charge of their skin health, drawing from the wisdom of the past while embracing the advancements of contemporary dermatology.

Comparative Analysis of Skin Care Regimens

In the realm of dermatological health care, the comparative analysis of skin care regimens is essential for health professionals and adults seeking to optimize skin health. Skin care regimens vary widely across cultures, influenced by factors such as environmental conditions, available resources, and traditional practices. By examining these diverse approaches, professionals can gain insights into effective strategies that may be adapted for various skin types and conditions, ultimately enhancing patient care and personal skin health management.

Natural remedies have gained traction as holistic treatments for various skin issues. Many cultures employ herbal solutions that have been passed down through generations. Ingredients such as aloe vera, chamomile, and calendula are frequently used to soothe irritated skin and promote healing. Analyzing these traditional practices alongside modern dermatological treatments can help professionals recommend a balanced approach that incorporates the potential benefits of natural remedies while ensuring the safety and efficacy of such treatments.

Another vital aspect of skin care regimens is tattoo aftercare, which requires specific guidelines to maintain skin integrity post-tattooing. The healing process of tattooed skin is critical, as improper aftercare can lead to infections and long-term skin damage. By comparing aftercare practices across different cultures, health professionals can identify commonalities and best practices that promote optimal healing. This not only aids in preserving the aesthetic quality of tattoos but also contributes to broader skin health.

Nutrition plays a significant role in skin health, impacting conditions such as acne, eczema, and signs of aging. A comparative analysis of dietary practices can reveal how different cultural approaches to nutrition influence skin health outcomes. For instance, diets rich in antioxidants, omega-3 fatty acids, and vitamins can enhance skin resilience and appearance. By integrating nutritional education into skin care regimens, health professionals can empower individuals to make informed dietary choices that support their skin health.

Finally, understanding the interplay between skin conditions and external factors, such as allergens and irritants, is crucial for effective skin care. A thorough examination of skin allergies and their triggers can inform the development of protective measures, including barrier creams. Additionally, health professionals should be equipped with first aid techniques for common skin injuries, ensuring they can provide immediate care and guidance. By synthesizing knowledge from various niches within dermatological health care, this comparative analysis serves as a foundation for developing comprehensive skin care regimens tailored to individual needs and cultural contexts.

Chapter 6: Skin Cancer Awareness and Prevention

Types of Skin Cancer and Risk Factors

Skin cancer is a significant public health concern, representing one of the most prevalent forms of cancer globally. The three primary types of skin cancer are basal cell carcinoma (BCC), squamous cell carcinoma (SCC), and melanoma. Basal cell carcinoma is the most common type, typically appearing as a small, shiny bump or a pink growth on sun-exposed areas, such as the face and neck. It arises from the basal cells in the epidermis and is usually slow-growing, making it less likely to metastasize. Squamous cell carcinoma, on the other hand, originates from the squamous cells in the skin and can manifest as a firm, red nodule or a flat lesion with a scaly, crusted surface. While SCC is more aggressive than BCC, it is still highly treatable when detected early. Melanoma, though less common, is the most dangerous form of skin cancer due to its ability to spread rapidly to other parts of the body. It often appears as an irregularly shaped mole or a change in an existing mole's appearance.

Understanding the risk factors associated with skin cancer is critical for effective prevention and early detection. Ultraviolet (UV) radiation from the sun is the primary risk factor, with excessive sun exposure leading to DNA damage in skin cells. Individuals with fair skin, light hair, and blue or green eyes are at a heightened risk due to lower levels of melanin, which provides some protection against UV damage. Other risk factors include a personal or family history of skin cancer, a weakened immune system, and the presence of numerous moles or atypical moles. Environmental factors, such as living in sunny climates or working in outdoor occupations, also contribute to increased risk. Furthermore, certain medications that suppress the immune system may elevate the likelihood of developing skin cancer.

In addition to these intrinsic and extrinsic risk factors, lifestyle choices play a significant role in skin health and cancer prevention. Smoking has been linked to an increased risk of squamous cell carcinoma, while excessive alcohol consumption can also negatively impact skin integrity and immune response. Moreover, poor dietary habits may compromise skin health, emphasizing the importance of a balanced diet rich in antioxidants, vitamins, and minerals. Nutritional strategies such as increasing the intake of fruits, vegetables, and omega-3 fatty acids can bolster skin resilience against environmental stressors and may aid in cancer prevention.

Education and awareness are paramount in combating skin cancer. Health professionals must emphasize the importance of regular skin checks and self-examinations, encouraging individuals to report any suspicious changes promptly. Protective measures against UV radiation, such as wearing broad-spectrum sunscreen, protective clothing, and seeking shade, should be reinforced. Additionally, public health campaigns that focus on skin cancer awareness can significantly impact community attitudes towards sun safety and early detection, ultimately leading to better health outcomes.

In conclusion, the multifaceted approach to understanding the types of skin cancer and their associated risk factors is essential for health professionals and individuals alike. By fostering awareness of the various forms of skin cancer, recognizing risk factors, and promoting preventative strategies, we can mitigate the incidence of skin cancer and enhance overall dermatological health. This knowledge empowers individuals to make informed decisions about their skin care, contributes to holistic health practices, and underscores the importance of integrating preventive measures into daily life.

Nutrition and Skin Cancer Prevention

Nutrition plays a pivotal role in skin health, influencing not only its appearance but also its resilience against diseases such as skin cancer. As health professionals and informed adults seek to understand the multifaceted relationship between dietary choices and dermatological outcomes, it becomes essential to explore how specific nutrients can bolster skin defenses. A well-balanced diet rich in antioxidants, vitamins, and minerals can mitigate the risk factors associated with skin cancer, emphasizing the importance of nutrition as a proactive approach to skin health.

Antioxidants, including vitamins C and E, are crucial in combating oxidative stress, a significant contributor to skin damage and cancer progression. Foods such as berries, nuts, and green leafy vegetables are abundant in these protective compounds. They neutralize free radicals, which can cause cellular damage and promote carcinogenesis. Moreover, a diet rich in carotenoids, found in fruits and vegetables like carrots, sweet potatoes, and spinach, may enhance skin health by providing additional protection against UV radiation, thereby reducing the likelihood of skin cancer development.

Omega-3 fatty acids, prevalent in fatty fish, flaxseeds, and walnuts, also play a vital role in maintaining skin integrity. These essential fats help regulate inflammatory processes within the body, potentially reducing the incidence of skin conditions that can predispose individuals to cancer. By incorporating omega-3-rich foods into their diets, individuals may not only improve their overall skin health but also reinforce their skin's natural defense mechanisms against harmful environmental factors.

In addition to specific nutrients, overall dietary patterns significantly influence skin cancer risk. Diets high in processed foods and sugars can lead to systemic inflammation and impaired immune function, both of which are linked to increased cancer susceptibility. A Mediterranean-style diet, characterized by whole grains, lean proteins, healthy fats, and abundant fruits and vegetables, has been associated with lower rates of various cancers, including skin cancer. Health professionals should advocate for such dietary patterns to enhance skin health and promote cancer prevention.

Finally, education on the importance of hydration cannot be overlooked in the context of skin health and cancer prevention. Adequate water intake supports skin elasticity and function, playing a crucial role in maintaining the skin barrier. Health professionals should encourage individuals to not only focus on the types of food consumed but also prioritize hydration as a fundamental component of their daily regimen. By integrating these nutritional strategies into their practice, health professionals can empower individuals to take control of their skin health and reduce the risk of skin cancer through informed dietary choices.

Protective Measures and Sun Safety

Protective measures and sun safety are critical components of dermatological health care, particularly in the prevention of skin damage and the promotion of overall skin integrity. As health professionals and adults navigate the complexities of skin care, understanding the multifaceted relationship between ultraviolet (UV) radiation and skin health becomes paramount. Both UVA and UVB rays can lead to various skin issues, including premature aging, sunburn, and an increased risk of skin cancer.

Effective protective measures must be implemented to mitigate these risks and promote healthy skin across diverse populations.

The foundation of sun safety lies in the consistent use of broad-spectrum sunscreen, which shields the skin from both UVA and UVB rays. Health professionals should emphasize the importance of selecting a sunscreen with an SPF of at least 30, applying it generously to all exposed skin, and reapplying every two hours—more frequently during water activities or excessive sweating. Additionally, it is essential to educate patients about the expiration dates of sunscreen and the significance of using products that are free from harmful chemicals. This knowledge empowers individuals to make informed choices, particularly in the context of natural remedies and holistic treatments that align with their values and cultural practices.

In addition to sunscreen, protective clothing serves as a vital component of sun safety. Long-sleeved shirts, wide-brimmed hats, and UV-blocking sunglasses not only provide physical barriers against UV radiation but also enhance the effectiveness of sunscreen. Health professionals should advocate for the use of UPF-rated clothing as a proactive measure, particularly for those with increased sensitivity to sunlight or a history of skin conditions. Awareness of the cultural significance of protective clothing can foster inclusivity in discussions about skin health, recognizing that different cultures may have unique approaches to sun safety that should be respected and integrated into care strategies.

The role of nutrition in bolstering skin health cannot be overlooked when discussing protective measures. A diet rich in antioxidants, vitamins, and minerals supports the skin's ability to repair itself and defend against environmental damage, including sun exposure. Health professionals should guide patients towards incorporating foods high in omega-3 fatty acids, vitamins C and E, and polyphenols, which can enhance the skin's resilience. Additionally, hydration plays a crucial role in maintaining skin elasticity and barrier function, further underscoring the interconnectedness of nutrition, skin health, and protective measures.

Lastly, skin cancer awareness and prevention strategies must be a cornerstone of any comprehensive dermatological health care plan. Regular skin examinations, self-monitoring for changes in moles or skin lesions, and education about the signs of skin cancer are essential in early detection and treatment. By promoting a culture of sun safety and protective measures, health professionals can significantly reduce the incidence of skin cancer and empower individuals to take charge of their skin health. Integrating these principles into practice not only enhances patient outcomes but also contributes to a broader understanding of how environmental factors and personal choices affect dermatological health across diverse populations.

Chapter 7: Managing Incontinence and Skin Care

Skin Damage Prevention Strategies

Skin damage can result from a variety of environmental factors, lifestyle choices, and underlying health conditions. For health professionals and informed adults, understanding and implementing effective prevention strategies is essential to maintaining skin integrity and overall health. This subchapter will explore comprehensive approaches to skin damage prevention, emphasizing the importance of holistic treatments, proper aftercare practices, and nutritional considerations, while also addressing the broader implications of skin health across different cultures.

Natural remedies for skin conditions often provide a foundational approach to skin health. Utilizing herbal solutions, such as aloe vera for its soothing properties or chamomile for its anti-inflammatory effects, can complement conventional treatments. These remedies can be particularly beneficial for individuals with sensitive skin or those seeking to minimize chemical exposure. Health professionals should encourage patients to explore these options while educating them on the importance of patch testing to avoid adverse reactions. Integrating holistic treatments into daily skincare routines can significantly enhance the skin's resilience against damage.

In the context of tattoo aftercare, maintaining skin health post-tattooing is crucial for preventing infections and ensuring proper healing. Professionals should advocate for a rigorous aftercare regimen that includes keeping the tattooed area clean, moisturized, and protected from excessive sun exposure. The use of barrier creams can be particularly effective in this regard, offering a protective layer that shields the skin from environmental aggressors while promoting healing. Educating clients about the importance of following aftercare instructions can lead to improved outcomes and enhanced skin integrity.

Nutrition plays a pivotal role in skin health, influencing everything from hydration to the skin's ability to repair itself. Diets rich in antioxidants, healthy fats, and vitamins can combat the effects of aging and environmental damage. Health professionals should emphasize the importance of a balanced diet that includes fruits, vegetables, whole grains, and lean proteins. Additionally, understanding the cultural differences in dietary practices and their impact on skin health can provide valuable insights for tailored recommendations. This holistic approach to nutrition allows for a more personalized care plan, ultimately leading to healthier skin.

Lastly, skin cancer awareness and prevention strategies must be at the forefront of skin health discussions. Education on the various types of skin cancer, their risk factors, and the importance of regular skin examinations is crucial for early detection and treatment. Professionals should also promote the use of sunscreen, protective clothing, and regular dermatological check-ups as essential components of skin health maintenance. By combining knowledge of skin types, cultural practices, and preventative measures, health professionals can empower individuals to take charge of their skin health and minimize the risk of damage, ensuring a more resilient and vibrant complexion.

Infection Control and Hygiene Practices

Infection control and hygiene practices are critical components of dermatological health care, especially in the context of maintaining skin integrity and preventing infections. For health professionals and adults alike, understanding the best practices for infection control can significantly impact overall skin health, particularly in scenarios involving natural remedies, post-tattoo care, and management of various skin conditions. The skin is not only the body's first line of defense against pathogens but also a sensitive organ that can be easily compromised by improper hygiene practices.

One of the foundational elements of effective infection control is the consistent application of proper hand hygiene. Health professionals should advocate for regular handwashing with soap and water, or the use of alcohol-based hand sanitizers, to eliminate harmful microorganisms that could potentially lead to skin infections. This practice is especially pertinent when dealing with open wounds, tattoos, or any skin treatment that could introduce bacteria. Additionally, adults should be educated on the importance of keeping their hands clean before applying any topical treatments or handling skin care products, particularly in the context of natural remedies and holistic approaches to skin health.

Furthermore, understanding the role of environmental factors in infection control is essential. Maintaining a clean environment not only supports individual hygiene but also reduces the risk of cross-contamination. This is particularly crucial in settings where skin health is a priority, such as tattoo parlors, dermatology clinics, and holistic health practices. Regularly disinfecting surfaces and ensuring that tools and equipment are sterilized can prevent the transmission of infections. For individuals managing skin conditions or recovering from procedures like tattooing, creating a clean space for healing can facilitate recovery and minimize the risk of complications.

Infection control practices extend beyond just hand hygiene and environmental cleanliness; they also encompass the use of appropriate skin care products. For instance, barrier creams can be an effective tool in protecting the skin from irritants and pathogens, especially for individuals managing incontinence or those in professions with high exposure to hazardous materials. Health professionals should guide patients in selecting barrier creams that suit their specific skin types and conditions, ensuring that these products are applied correctly to maximize their protective effects. This consideration is particularly relevant for individuals with sensitive skin or those recovering from allergic reactions.

Lastly, patient education on recognizing signs of infection and understanding when to seek medical advice is paramount. Adults should be informed about the symptoms indicating a potential infection, such as increased redness, swelling, or discharge from a wound. In cases of skin injuries or conditions exacerbated by allergies, timely intervention can prevent further complications and promote better skin health. By integrating comprehensive infection control and hygiene practices into dermatological care, health professionals can significantly enhance patient outcomes, fostering a preventative approach to skin health that encompasses education, awareness, and effective management strategies.

The Role of Nutrition in Skin Resilience

The health and appearance of the skin are intrinsically linked to nutritional intake, making diet a crucial factor in skin resilience. Nutrients such as vitamins, minerals, and antioxidants play a vital role in maintaining skin integrity and function. For health professionals, understanding the biochemical interactions between nutrition and the skin can enhance the efficacy of treatment plans, especially for patients dealing with skin conditions or post-tattoo care. A well-rounded diet not only supports the skin's barrier function but also mitigates signs of aging and promotes a radiant complexion.

Key nutrients for skin health include vitamins A, C, and E, which are known for their antioxidant properties. Vitamin A, essential for skin cell production and repair, can be sourced from foods like carrots and sweet potatoes. Vitamin C is critical for collagen synthesis, helping to maintain skin structure and elasticity, and can be found in citrus fruits and leafy greens. Vitamin E acts as a protector against oxidative stress, often accumulated through environmental exposure. This triad of vitamins underscores the importance of a varied diet rich in fruits and vegetables, which health professionals should advocate for their patients.

In addition to vitamins, essential fatty acids, particularly omega-3 and omega-6, are fundamental in maintaining skin hydration and elasticity. These fatty acids can be obtained from sources such as fish, flaxseeds, and walnuts. They work to strengthen the skin's lipid barrier, preventing trans-epidermal water loss and protecting against inflammatory skin conditions. For individuals with compromised skin barriers, including those recovering from tattoos or managing chronic skin conditions, incorporating these healthy fats can significantly improve skin resilience.

Moreover, hydration plays a pivotal role in skin health. Water is essential for maintaining skin turgor and preventing dryness, which can lead to irritation and exacerbate skin issues. Health professionals should emphasize the importance of adequate water intake alongside dietary recommendations, as hydration from both food and beverages is vital. Foods with high water content, such as cucumbers, oranges, and broths, can contribute to overall hydration and enhance skin appearance.

Lastly, the impact of dietary habits extends beyond evident skin conditions; it also encompasses broader health implications. A diet high in processed foods, sugars, and unhealthy fats can lead to inflammatory responses, potentially aggravating skin issues and accelerating aging. By promoting a diet that emphasizes whole foods and nutritional balance, health professionals can foster not only improved skin resilience but also overall health and well-being in their patients. The integration of nutritional education into dermatological health care will empower individuals to make informed dietary choices that support their skin's needs across various contexts, from managing skin conditions to post-tattoo care.

Chapter 8: Barrier Creams and Their Effectiveness

Overview of Barrier Creams and Their Uses

Barrier creams play a crucial role in dermatological health care by providing a protective layer on the skin, shielding it from irritants, moisture, and environmental stressors. These creams are formulated with occlusive agents that form a physical barrier, which can help prevent skin damage and promote healing in various contexts. Health professionals often recommend barrier creams not only for general skin protection but also for specific applications such as tattoo aftercare, managing incontinence, and protecting the skin in occupational settings. Understanding the composition and effectiveness of these products is essential for both practitioners and patients to make informed decisions regarding skin care.

In the realm of tattoo aftercare, the use of barrier creams is particularly significant. Newly tattooed skin is susceptible to infection and irritation, making it imperative to apply a product that not only protects but also allows for the skin's natural healing processes. Barrier creams designed for this purpose often contain ingredients that are both soothing and hydrating, helping to maintain skin integrity while minimizing the risk of adverse reactions. By educating clients on the proper use of these creams, health professionals can significantly enhance the healing experience and ensure the longevity of the tattoo.

Cultural considerations also play a vital role in the use of barrier creams. Different skin types across cultures may respond differently to various formulations. For instance, individuals with darker skin may experience distinct challenges with moisture retention and hyperpigmentation, influencing the types of barrier creams that are most effective for them. Recognizing these differences is essential for health professionals to provide personalized care and recommendations, fostering an inclusive approach to dermatological health that respects the diversity of skin types and the unique needs of various populations.

Nutrition is another critical factor that intersects with the effectiveness of barrier creams. A diet rich in vitamins, minerals, and antioxidants can enhance skin health, making the skin more resilient to external irritants. Health professionals should encourage patients to adopt a holistic approach that combines the use of barrier creams with proper nutritional practices. This synergy not only aids in skin protection but also supports overall skin health and can mitigate some underlying conditions that may compromise the skin's barrier function.

Finally, it is important to highlight the role of barrier creams in managing specific skin conditions, such as those related to incontinence. These creams can prevent skin breakdown and irritation caused by prolonged exposure to moisture and irritants. By understanding the various types of barrier creams and their specific applications, health professionals can develop effective strategies to protect vulnerable skin areas, ultimately enhancing patient outcomes and promoting a proactive approach to dermatological health care. Barrier creams, when chosen and applied correctly, can provide invaluable support in maintaining skin integrity across various contexts and conditions.

Efficacy of Barrier Creams in Various Conditions

Efficacy of barrier creams in various conditions is an essential topic for healthcare professionals and adults seeking to enhance their understanding of skin protection strategies. Barrier creams serve as a vital line of defense against external irritants and environmental factors that can compromise skin integrity. These formulations create a physical barrier on the skin's surface, which can mitigate the adverse effects of moisture, friction, and harmful substances. The effectiveness of these creams varies depending on their ingredients, application methods, and the specific skin conditions being addressed.

In clinical settings, barrier creams are frequently utilized for patients with compromised skin barriers, such as those suffering from incontinence or dermatitis. For individuals experiencing incontinence, barrier creams can prevent maceration and skin breakdown by providing a protective layer against moisture. Studies have demonstrated that regular application of these creams significantly reduces the incidence of pressure ulcers and dermatitis in affected populations. Furthermore, the incorporation of natural ingredients, such as aloe vera and calendula, has shown promising results in enhancing skin healing and reducing inflammation.

Barrier creams also play a critical role in tattoo aftercare, where maintaining skin integrity is paramount for optimal healing. The application of these creams can help prevent irritation from external contaminants and excessive moisture, which may lead to complications during the healing process. Health professionals often recommend barrier creams containing zinc oxide or titanium dioxide for their protective properties and ability to soothe inflamed skin. As tattoos become increasingly popular, understanding the efficacy of barrier creams in this context is essential for promoting safe and healthy tattoo practices.

The relationship between nutrition and skin health cannot be overlooked when discussing the efficacy of barrier creams. A diet rich in antioxidants, vitamins, and essential fatty acids can enhance the skin's natural barrier function, thereby complementing the protective effects of topical treatments. Nutritional factors can influence the skin's response to irritants and its overall resilience, suggesting that a holistic approach that includes both dietary considerations and the use of barrier creams is vital for optimal skin health. Healthcare professionals should encourage patients to adopt a balanced diet alongside appropriate topical interventions.

Lastly, awareness of allergic reactions and their impact on skin health underscores the importance of selecting barrier creams tailored to individual skin types and conditions. Many conventional products contain potential allergens that could exacerbate existing skin issues or lead to new reactions. Therefore, it is crucial for practitioners to guide patients in choosing hypoallergenic options that contain minimal irritants. By understanding the unique needs of diverse skin types across cultures and the potential risks associated with various formulations, health professionals can better support individuals in managing their skin health effectively.

Choosing the Right Barrier Cream

Choosing the right barrier cream is a critical aspect of maintaining skin health and preventing damage, particularly in specific contexts such as tattoo aftercare, managing incontinence, and preventing skin reactions due to allergies. Barrier creams serve as a protective layer that can help shield the skin from irritants, moisture, and external contaminants. Given the diverse needs of individuals, health professionals must consider various factors, including skin type, underlying conditions, and the specific environmental challenges faced by the patient. This subchapter aims to guide health professionals and informed adults in selecting the most suitable barrier cream for their unique requirements.

When evaluating barrier creams, it is essential to understand the formulation and ingredients that comprise these products. Natural remedies and holistic treatments have gained popularity, with many barrier creams incorporating herbal solutions known for their skin-soothing properties. Ingredients like aloe vera, calendula, and chamomile not only offer protective benefits but also promote healing and hydration. Health professionals should be well-versed in these ingredients, as they can provide valuable recommendations tailored to the individual's skin type and condition, ensuring optimal results while minimizing the risk of adverse reactions.

The context in which a barrier cream will be used significantly influences the selection process. For instance, in tattoo aftercare, a barrier cream that is non-comedogenic and free from irritating fragrances is essential to maintain skin integrity while promoting healing. Similarly, for individuals managing incontinence, barrier creams that provide long-lasting protection against moisture and friction are paramount. Professionals should conduct thorough assessments of the patient's lifestyle and specific challenges to recommend barrier creams that effectively address their needs while maintaining skin health.

Cultural considerations also play a vital role in choosing the right barrier cream. Different skin types across various cultures may respond differently to particular ingredients or formulations. Understanding these nuances enables health professionals to recommend products that align with cultural practices and preferences. Additionally, knowledge of how nutrition impacts skin health can inform recommendations, as a well-balanced diet can enhance the skin's resilience, potentially affecting the efficacy of barrier creams.

In conclusion, selecting the appropriate barrier cream requires a comprehensive understanding of the patient's skin type, environmental factors, and cultural considerations. Health professionals should leverage their expertise in dermatological health to guide individuals toward products that not only protect the skin but also support its overall integrity and resilience. Through informed choices, patients can achieve better skin health outcomes, whether it be in the context of tattoo care, managing skin conditions, or preventing irritations and allergies.

Chapter 9: First Aid Techniques for Common Skin Injuries

Treating Blisters and Minor Burns

Blisters and minor burns are common skin injuries that can occur in a variety of situations, from everyday activities to more specialized contexts such as tattoo aftercare. Understanding the appropriate treatment for these injuries is crucial for health professionals and adults alike, as improper care can lead to complications such as infection or prolonged discomfort. This subchapter will explore effective treatment strategies using both conventional and natural remedies, emphasizing the importance of holistic approaches in dermatological health care.

The initial step in treating blisters involves proper assessment. Blisters, which are small pockets of fluid that form between the skin layers, can arise from friction, heat, or chemical exposure. For minor burns, characterized by skin redness, pain, and swelling, immediate cooling of the affected area is essential. Running cool (not cold) water over the burn for 10 to 20 minutes helps to alleviate pain and prevent further tissue damage. In the case of blisters, it is generally advised to avoid popping them, as the intact skin serves as a protective barrier against infection. Instead, cover the blister with a sterile, non-adhesive bandage to promote healing.

Natural remedies can complement conventional treatments for blisters and burns. Aloe vera, with its anti-inflammatory and hydrating properties, is widely recognized for its ability to soothe burned skin and accelerate healing. Applying pure aloe vera gel directly to the affected area can provide relief and support skin regeneration. Other herbal solutions, such as calendula and chamomile, have also shown efficacy in reducing inflammation and promoting skin repair. These holistic treatments can be particularly appealing to those seeking alternatives to pharmaceutical interventions, especially in the context of tattoo aftercare, where skin integrity is paramount.

Nutrition plays a pivotal role in skin health and healing. A well-balanced diet rich in vitamins A, C, and E, as well as omega-3 fatty acids, can enhance the skin's resilience and repair mechanisms. Foods such as leafy greens, nuts, seeds, and fatty fish contribute essential nutrients that support skin regeneration, making them valuable additions to the diet of individuals prone to blisters and burns. Encouraging patients and clients to adopt a nutrient-dense diet can foster better overall skin health and mitigate the risk of injuries related to skin integrity.

Preventive measures are also crucial in the management of blisters and minor burns. Educating individuals about appropriate protective gear during high-risk activities, such as cooking or engaging in manual labor, can significantly reduce the likelihood of injury. Additionally, understanding the impact of allergic reactions on skin health is vital, as certain individuals may be more susceptible to developing blisters or burns due to sensitivities or underlying skin conditions. By combining knowledge of first aid techniques, natural remedies, and nutritional strategies, health professionals can provide comprehensive care that addresses both immediate treatment and long-term skin health.

Proper Care for Cuts and Scrapes

Proper care for cuts and scrapes is an essential aspect of dermatological health that not only promotes healing but also mitigates the risk of infection and scarring. For health professionals and adults alike, understanding the appropriate methods for managing these common skin injuries can significantly enhance recovery outcomes. The initial approach to treating cuts and scrapes involves a series of systematic steps that prioritize cleanliness and protection of the affected area. By adopting evidence-based practices, individuals can ensure that they are providing optimal care, which is particularly important in the context of holistic health approaches that emphasize natural remedies.

The first step in caring for a cut or scrape is to cleanse the wound thoroughly. This involves rinsing the area with clean water to remove any debris and contaminants. For deeper wounds, saline solutions can be beneficial as they help minimize irritation. It is advisable to avoid using hydrogen peroxide or alcohol directly on the wound, as these agents can damage healthy tissue and prolong the healing process. Instead, gentle soap and water are recommended for initial cleansing. Following this, the application of a natural antiseptic, such as honey or tea tree oil, may serve to enhance healing due to their antibacterial properties, aligning with holistic treatment principles.

Once the wound is cleansed and treated, proper dressing is crucial in protecting it from further injury and infection. A sterile bandage or dressing should be applied, ensuring that it is secure but not overly tight, allowing for adequate circulation. Regularly changing the dressing is essential to keep the area clean and monitor for any signs of infection, such as increased redness, swelling, or discharge. In the context of tattoo aftercare, similar principles apply, where maintaining cleanliness and moisture balance can significantly impact the healing of the skin post-tattooing.

Nutrition plays a vital role in the body's healing process, including the recovery of cuts and scrapes. A diet rich in vitamins A, C, and E, along with adequate protein intake, supports skin repair and regeneration. Health professionals should encourage individuals to consume foods that promote collagen synthesis and reduce inflammation, such as leafy greens, citrus fruits, nuts, and fatty fish. This holistic approach not only aids in wound healing but also contributes to overall skin health, addressing other skin conditions effectively.

Lastly, awareness of potential allergic reactions and skin sensitivities is critical when caring for cuts and scrapes. Individuals with known allergies should be cautious about the products used on their skin during the healing process. Barrier creams can provide an additional layer of protection, particularly in environments where exposure to irritants or moisture is a concern. By integrating these comprehensive care strategies, health professionals and adults can enhance their understanding of proper wound management, ensuring effective healing and the maintenance of skin integrity in various contexts.

When to Seek Professional Medical Help

When it comes to dermatological health, understanding when to seek professional medical help is crucial for effective treatment and prevention of complications. While many skin conditions can be managed through natural remedies and at-home care, there are circumstances where professional intervention becomes necessary. Recognizing the signs that warrant a visit to a healthcare provider is essential, particularly for health professionals who guide patients and adults who are proactive about their skin health. This subchapter outlines key indicators that suggest the need for professional assistance, ensuring that individuals can make informed decisions about their dermatological care.

The first indicator involves persistent or worsening symptoms that do not respond to over-the-counter treatments or home remedies. Many skin issues, such as eczema, psoriasis, or acne, can initially be addressed through holistic approaches or topical applications. However, if symptoms such as intense itching, significant inflammation, or widespread lesions continue to escalate despite these measures, it is imperative to consult a dermatologist. Persistent symptoms may indicate an underlying condition that requires more specialized treatment, which can prevent further complications, including infections or scarring.

Another critical factor is the presence of systemic symptoms accompanying skin issues. Signs such as fever, fatigue, or unexplained weight loss can indicate that a skin condition is part of a broader systemic illness. For example, conditions like lupus or other autoimmune diseases can manifest through dermatological symptoms. Health professionals must be vigilant in assessing these signs, as timely intervention can lead to better health outcomes. Recognizing the interconnectedness of skin health and overall well-being can guide patients to seek appropriate care when necessary.

Skin cancer awareness is another area where professional guidance is indispensable. Regular self-examinations for new or changing moles, as well as understanding the risk factors associated with various types of skin cancer, can empower individuals to take charge of their skin health. However, any suspicious changes—such as asymmetry, irregular borders, or variations in color—should prompt an immediate consultation with a healthcare provider. Early detection is critical in managing skin cancer effectively, and health professionals play a vital role in educating patients about the importance of monitoring their skin.

In addition to the aforementioned indicators, individuals managing chronic conditions, such as incontinence, should seek professional help to address skin integrity and prevent complications. Prolonged exposure to moisture can lead to skin breakdown and infections, necessitating the use of specialized barrier creams and other preventive measures. A healthcare provider can offer tailored advice and interventions that align with each patient's unique needs, ensuring that skin health is maintained even in challenging circumstances.

Understanding when to seek professional medical help is a fundamental aspect of effective dermatological health care. By recognizing persistent symptoms, systemic indicators, risks associated with skin cancer, and challenges related to chronic conditions, both health professionals and adults can take proactive steps toward safeguarding their skin health. This knowledge not only enhances individual well-being but also fosters a culture of informed decision-making in dermatological care.

Chapter 10: The Impact of Allergic Reactions on Skin

Common Allergens and Their Effects on the Skin

Common allergens can significantly impact skin health, eliciting a range of reactions that vary in severity among individuals. Common sources of allergens include substances found in everyday environments such as pollen, pet dander, certain foods, and various chemicals in skincare and cosmetic products. Exposure to these allergens can lead to dermatological conditions like contact dermatitis, urticaria (hives), and other forms of eczema, which can cause discomfort, inflammation, and long-term skin damage if left untreated. Understanding the nature of these allergens and their effects is crucial for health professionals and adults alike, particularly in the context of holistic skin care.

One of the most prevalent allergens is nickel, commonly found in jewelry, clothing fasteners, and certain types of cosmetics. Individuals with nickel sensitivity may experience localized dermatitis characterized by redness, itching, and blistering upon contact. It is essential for health professionals to educate patients on identifying nickel-containing products and suggest alternatives. Similarly, fragrances—both synthetic and natural—can trigger allergic reactions. These reactions may manifest as rashes or exacerbation of pre-existing conditions like eczema, necessitating a careful review of product ingredients for those with sensitive skin.

Another significant class of allergens is derived from common food items, particularly in individuals with atopic dermatitis. Foods such as peanuts, tree nuts, dairy, and gluten can provoke systemic reactions that may manifest as skin issues, including rashes and severe itching. The relationship between diet and skin health underscores the importance of a holistic approach to dermatological care. Health professionals should consider incorporating dietary assessments and recommendations into their practice, promoting a better understanding of how nutrition influences skin conditions.

Pet dander and pollen are also notable allergens that can contribute to skin problems. For instance, individuals with allergic rhinitis may experience skin reactions such as itchiness or hives as part of their overall allergic response. This phenomenon highlights the interconnectedness of environmental factors and skin health. Effective management strategies could include allergy testing, environmental control measures, and appropriate skin care regimens designed to soothe and protect the skin barrier, thereby minimizing allergic responses.

In conclusion, recognizing common allergens and their effects on the skin is vital for both health professionals and adults seeking to maintain optimal skin health. A comprehensive understanding of allergens, their sources, and their impact on the skin can inform better patient education and self-care practices. By adopting a holistic approach that includes dietary considerations, environmental awareness, and appropriate skincare, individuals can effectively manage allergic reactions and promote healthier skin outcomes. This knowledge is particularly relevant for those navigating the complexities of skin health across various cultural and personal contexts, emphasizing the need for tailored solutions in dermatological care.

Symptoms and Diagnosis of Skin Allergies

Skin allergies manifest through a variety of symptoms that can range from mild irritation to severe reactions. Common indicators include redness, itching, swelling, and the development of rashes or hives. These reactions can occur shortly after exposure to an allergen or may take time to develop, complicating the identification of triggers. In some cases, individuals may experience dermatitis, which presents as flaky, dry skin that can become crusty or weepy. Recognizing these symptoms is crucial for health professionals to provide appropriate interventions and educate patients about managing their skin health.

Diagnosis of skin allergies typically begins with a comprehensive patient history and physical examination. Health professionals should gather detailed information about the patient's symptoms, including onset, duration, and any potential exposure to allergens. For a confirmed diagnosis, dermatologists often utilize patch testing, which involves applying small amounts of various allergens to the skin to observe reactions over a few days. This method is particularly effective in identifying contact allergens that may not be immediately apparent. Blood tests may also be employed to detect specific antibodies related to allergic reactions, although these are less commonly used for skin allergies than patch tests.

It is essential for health professionals to differentiate between skin allergies and other dermatological conditions, such as eczema or psoriasis, which may present with similar symptoms. A thorough understanding of the patient's medical history and potential environmental triggers is critical in this process. Moreover, understanding cultural nuances in skin health can aid in diagnosis, as certain skin types may exhibit varying responses to allergens. This comparative analysis can enhance diagnostic accuracy and lead to more tailored treatment plans that respect cultural practices and beliefs.

Once a diagnosis is established, management strategies can be developed. Treatment often involves the identification and avoidance of allergens, which may require lifestyle modifications. Topical treatments, such as corticosteroids or antihistamines, can provide symptomatic relief. In addition, natural remedies and holistic treatments are gaining traction among patients seeking alternatives to conventional therapies. Health professionals should be prepared to discuss the efficacy and safety of herbal solutions, ensuring that patients are well-informed about potential interactions with prescribed medications.

Lastly, education plays a vital role in the management of skin allergies. Health professionals must equip patients with knowledge about their conditions, emphasizing the importance of protective measures, such as using barrier creams and adopting a suitable skincare regimen. Additionally, discussions about the role of nutrition in skin health can be beneficial, as certain dietary choices can influence skin reactions. By fostering an understanding of the relationship between lifestyle and skin health, professionals can empower individuals to take proactive steps in managing their skin allergies while maintaining overall wellness.

Treatment Options and Nutritional Considerations

In the realm of dermatological health, the intersection of treatment options and nutritional considerations plays a pivotal role in achieving optimal skin health. Professionals in this field must recognize the diverse array of holistic treatments and herbal solutions available for various skin conditions. These natural remedies, often derived from traditional practices, can complement conventional treatments and provide patients with alternatives that align with their personal health philosophies. By understanding the efficacy and safety of these remedies, health professionals can guide patients toward informed choices that enhance skin health while minimizing potential adverse effects.

Nutrition is equally critical in maintaining skin integrity and addressing specific dermatological issues. Recent research underscores the connection between diet and skin health, revealing that certain nutrients can significantly impact the appearance and functionality of the skin. For instance, vitamins A, C, and E, along with omega-3 fatty acids, play essential roles in skin repair and rejuvenation. Health professionals should encourage their patients to adopt a balanced diet rich in these nutrients, as well as antioxidants found in fruits and vegetables, to combat oxidative stress and promote a vibrant complexion. Additionally, understanding individual dietary needs based on skin type and conditions is crucial for tailoring nutritional advice.

Post-tattoo care is another area where treatment options and nutritional considerations intersect. Tattoo aftercare requires a comprehensive approach to maintain skin health and integrity during the healing process. Professionals should emphasize the importance of keeping the tattooed area clean and moisturized, while also recommending barrier creams that can protect the skin from external irritants. Furthermore, nutritional support, such as adequate hydration and a diet rich in vitamins and minerals, can facilitate the healing process and reduce the risk of complications. Educating clients about these aspects can enhance their aftercare experience and contribute to the longevity of their tattoos.

Cultural perspectives on skin health also warrant examination, particularly regarding beauty practices and their implications for treatment options. Different skin types across cultures may respond variably to certain treatments, necessitating an understanding of these differences in practice. By exploring and respecting diverse beauty ideals and skincare rituals, health professionals can offer more culturally competent care. This understanding fosters a more inclusive approach to dermatological health, allowing for individualized treatment plans that resonate with patients from various backgrounds.

Lastly, awareness of skin cancer and its prevention should be a fundamental part of conversations about treatment options. Educating patients about the types of skin cancer, associated risk factors, and protective measures is essential for early detection and intervention. Professionals must also consider the role of barrier creams in providing an additional layer of protection against harmful UV rays. As part of a comprehensive skin health strategy, the integration of nutritional considerations, holistic remedies, and preventive education can empower patients to take charge of their skin health, ultimately leading to better outcomes and enhanced quality of life.

Chapter 11: Makeup and Skin Health

The Relationship Between Cosmetics and Skin Conditions

The relationship between cosmetics and skin conditions is a multifaceted topic that warrants careful consideration, especially for health professionals and adults navigating their skincare choices. Cosmetics can serve as both a source of enhancement and a potential irritant. Understanding the composition of cosmetic products and their interactions with various skin types is crucial in preventing exacerbations of existing skin conditions and promoting overall skin health. This subchapter aims to elucidate the intricate dynamics between cosmetic use and skin integrity, offering insights into how to make informed choices in the realm of skincare.

Cosmetic products are often formulated with an array of ingredients, some of which can provoke allergic reactions or irritate sensitive skin. Common allergens include fragrances, preservatives, and certain colorants, which can lead to conditions such as contact dermatitis or exacerbation of eczema. Health professionals must be vigilant in identifying these irritants and advising patients on ingredient lists. Furthermore, the role of non-comedogenic products becomes essential for individuals with acne-prone skin, as the use of heavy or occlusive cosmetics can lead to clogged pores and subsequent breakouts.

The cultural context surrounding cosmetics also plays a significant role in shaping skin health practices. Across different cultures, beauty standards and cosmetic usage vary widely, influencing how individuals care for their skin. In some cultures, the use of natural and herbal remedies is prevalent, often considered more suitable for maintaining skin health. For health professionals, understanding these cultural differences can facilitate more personalized and effective treatment plans, particularly when addressing skin conditions that may be influenced by cosmetic use.

Nutrition is another critical factor that interplays with both cosmetics and skin health. The skin is a reflection of overall health, and dietary choices can significantly impact its appearance and condition. Health professionals should encourage patients to consider the synergy between what they apply topically and what they consume. A diet rich in antioxidants, vitamins, and healthy fats can bolster the skin's resilience, potentially mitigating some adverse effects of cosmetic use. Educating patients about the relationship between nutrition and skin health can empower them to make holistic choices that nurture their skin from both inside and out.

In conclusion, the intersection of cosmetics and skin conditions is a complex landscape that necessitates a thorough understanding of product formulations, cultural influences, and nutritional impacts. Health professionals play a pivotal role in guiding individuals towards safe and effective cosmetic choices that align with their skin health needs. By fostering awareness of potential irritants, promoting culturally sensitive practices, and emphasizing the importance of nutrition, practitioners can enhance the dermatological health of their patients while minimizing the risks associated with cosmetic use.

Tips for Choosing Skin-Friendly Makeup Products

Choosing skin-friendly makeup products is essential for maintaining overall skin health, particularly for individuals with specific skin conditions or sensitivities. As health professionals and informed adults increasingly recognize the intricate connection between cosmetics and dermatological wellbeing, it becomes imperative to consider various factors when selecting makeup. This subchapter will provide practical tips that prioritize skin health without compromising aesthetic preferences.

First and foremost, understanding skin type is crucial in selecting appropriate makeup products. Different skin types—oily, dry, sensitive, combination, and normal—require different formulations to avoid exacerbating existing conditions. For instance, those with oily or acne-prone skin should opt for non-comedogenic products that do not clog pores. Conversely, individuals with dry skin may benefit from hydrating formulations containing ingredients like hyaluronic acid or glycerin. Tailoring makeup choices to one's specific skin type not only enhances the overall appearance but also minimizes the risk of adverse reactions.

Another important consideration is ingredient transparency. Health professionals should encourage patients to read labels carefully and be aware of harmful additives such as parabens, sulfates, and synthetic fragrances, which can trigger allergic reactions or irritate sensitive skin. Instead, look for products with natural and organic ingredients, which are often gentler on the skin. Ingredients like aloe vera, chamomile, and green tea extract not only provide soothing benefits but also support the skin's natural barrier, promoting healthier skin over time.

Additionally, it is essential to consider the formulation and texture of makeup products. Cream-based products may be more suitable for dry or mature skin, offering hydration and a dewy finish, while powder formulations can be better for oily skin, helping to control shine. Moreover, opting for mineral-based makeup can provide an added layer of protection against environmental aggressors. These products often contain zinc oxide or titanium dioxide, which can act as physical sunscreens, offering additional protection against UV damage—a critical factor in skin cancer prevention.

Lastly, maintaining proper hygiene and application techniques can significantly impact skin health. Health professionals should advise patients to regularly clean makeup brushes and applicators to prevent the buildup of bacteria, which can lead to breakouts and infections. Furthermore, encouraging the practice of patch testing new products on a small area of skin can help identify potential allergic reactions before widespread application. By fostering a holistic approach that combines informed product selection with safe usage practices, individuals can enjoy the benefits of makeup while safeguarding their skin's integrity and health.

Caring for Sensitive Skin in a Cosmetic Context

Caring for sensitive skin in a cosmetic context requires an understanding of both the skin's unique characteristics and the potential impact of various cosmetic products. Sensitive skin is often more reactive to environmental factors, cosmetic ingredients, and even stress. Health professionals must educate their clients about the importance of identifying specific triggers, which can range from harsh chemicals in makeup to allergens in skincare products. By recognizing these triggers, individuals can take proactive steps to mitigate reactions and maintain skin integrity, ultimately enhancing their overall dermatological health.

When selecting cosmetic products for sensitive skin, it is essential to prioritize formulations that are hypoallergenic, fragrance-free, and devoid of common irritants. Many conventional cosmetics contain synthetic fragrances, preservatives, and alcohol, which can exacerbate sensitivity. From a holistic perspective, health professionals can guide clients toward natural remedies, such as plant-based oils and botanical extracts, which often provide soothing and nourishing properties without the harsh side effects associated with synthetic ingredients. Emphasizing the use of gentle formulations can help individuals with sensitive skin experience a more pleasant cosmetic application process.

Moreover, the role of nutrition in skin health cannot be overstated, particularly for individuals with sensitive skin. A diet rich in antioxidants, omega-3 fatty acids, and vitamins A, C, and E can promote a strong skin barrier and reduce inflammation. Health professionals should encourage their clients to consider dietary adjustments as part of their skincare routine. Incorporating foods such as fatty fish, nuts, and a variety of fruits and vegetables can contribute positively to skin resilience, thus enhancing the overall effectiveness of cosmetic products applied to sensitive areas.

Additionally, understanding the cultural context of sensitive skin care is vital for health professionals. Various cultures have unique beauty practices and remedies that cater to different skin types and sensitivities. By exploring these diverse approaches, practitioners can gain insights into alternative treatments and strategies that may benefit their clients. This comparative analysis not only broadens the knowledge base of health professionals but also fosters a more inclusive approach to skincare, recognizing the diverse needs of individuals from different backgrounds.

Finally, the importance of education in managing sensitive skin cannot be understated. Health professionals should provide clients with clear guidelines on proper skincare routines, including the use of barrier creams to protect against irritants and the importance of patch testing new products. By equipping individuals with the knowledge to make informed choices about their cosmetics, practitioners can empower them to maintain their skin health effectively. This comprehensive approach to caring for sensitive skin ensures that individuals can enjoy the benefits of cosmetics without compromising their dermatological health.

Chapter 12: Conclusion and Future Perspectives

Integrating Nutrition and Skin Care

The relationship between nutrition and skin health is a critical area of study that increasingly informs dermatological practices. As health professionals recognize the complexity of skin conditions, there is a growing emphasis on the role that diet plays in maintaining skin integrity and addressing various dermatological issues. Nutrients such as vitamins, minerals, and fatty acids have been shown to influence skin hydration, elasticity, and overall appearance. By integrating nutritional considerations into dermatological care, professionals can offer a more holistic approach that not only treats symptoms but also promotes long-term skin health.

Research indicates that certain dietary components can significantly affect skin conditions. For instance, omega-3 fatty acids, found in fish and flaxseeds, possess anti-inflammatory properties that can alleviate conditions like acne and eczema. Antioxidant-rich foods, including fruits and vegetables, provide essential protection against oxidative stress, which is a contributing factor to skin aging and damage. Moreover, hydration plays a pivotal role in maintaining skin moisture and elasticity. Encouraging patients to consume adequate water and hydrating foods can enhance skin texture and resilience, making it an essential aspect of any skin care regimen.

The integration of nutrition into skin care becomes particularly vital when considering cultural variations in dietary practices. Different cultural backgrounds may influence the types of foods individuals consume, which in turn affects their skin health. For example, the

Mediterranean diet, rich in fruits, vegetables, whole grains, and healthy fats, is often associated with lower incidents of skin diseases. Understanding these cultural nuances enables health professionals to tailor dietary recommendations that resonate with diverse patient populations, enhancing the effectiveness of treatment plans.

Furthermore, the post-tattoo care process underscores the importance of nutrition in skin recovery. After tattooing, the skin requires optimal nutrients to heal effectively and maintain integrity. A diet rich in vitamins A and C, along with zinc, can support the healing process and minimize complications such as infections or scarring. Health professionals should educate their clients on the importance of nutrition in tattoo aftercare, emphasizing foods that promote skin repair and overall health as part of their recovery protocol.

In conclusion, integrating nutrition with skin care offers a comprehensive approach to dermatological health that extends beyond topical treatments. By recognizing the profound impact that dietary choices have on skin conditions, aging, and recovery, health professionals can provide a more holistic framework for patient care. This integration not only empowers individuals to make informed decisions about their diets but also fosters a proactive stance toward maintaining skin health across various stages of life. As the field of dermatology continues to evolve, the synergy between nutrition and skin care will undoubtedly play a pivotal role in shaping future practices and recommendations.

Emerging Research in Dermatological Health

Emerging research in dermatological health is shedding light on various aspects of skin care, emphasizing a holistic approach that encompasses natural remedies, nutritional influences, and culturally specific practices. This evolving field seeks to integrate traditional knowledge with contemporary scientific understanding, offering healthcare professionals and adults a comprehensive framework for managing skin conditions. The exploration of natural remedies for skin issues, for example, has garnered attention, as studies increasingly demonstrate the efficacy of herbal solutions and holistic treatments. This growing body of evidence encourages practitioners to consider alternative therapies alongside conventional dermatological practices, ultimately enhancing patient outcomes.

Tattoo aftercare represents another critical area of emerging research, as the popularity of body art continues to rise. Investigations into the best practices for maintaining skin integrity following tattooing reveal the importance of specific aftercare routines. Research has indicated that appropriate moisturizing and the use of barrier creams can significantly reduce the risk of infections and promote healing. Furthermore, understanding the skin's response to tattoo ink can lead to improved guidelines for both artists and clients, ensuring that the aesthetic benefits of tattoos do not compromise skin health.

The comparative analysis of skin types across cultures is an essential aspect of dermatological research that highlights the diverse beauty practices that reflect varying genetic backgrounds and environmental factors. Emerging studies suggest that cultural perspectives on skin health influence not only cosmetic choices but also the prevalence of certain dermatological conditions. By examining these cultural practices, health professionals can develop more effective, culturally sensitive treatment plans that resonate with diverse populations. This research ultimately advocates for a more inclusive approach to dermatological health care that recognizes and respects the unique needs of individuals from different backgrounds.

Nutrition's role in skin health is another significant focus of contemporary research, with findings indicating that dietary choices directly impact skin conditions, aging, and overall beauty. Emerging evidence suggests that specific nutrients, such as antioxidants, omega-3 fatty acids, and vitamins, play a critical role in maintaining skin elasticity and combating oxidative stress. Healthcare professionals are encouraged to integrate dietary assessments into their dermatological evaluations, emphasizing the importance of a balanced diet in promoting skin health. As the relationship between nutrition and dermatological conditions becomes clearer, practitioners can guide patients toward dietary modifications that enhance skin resilience.

Finally, the growing awareness of skin cancer underscores the need for education on prevention, risk factors, and protective measures. Research highlights the importance of early detection and the role of sunscreen and protective clothing in reducing skin cancer risks. Additionally, new insights into the impact of genetic predispositions and environmental exposures provide a more nuanced understanding of skin cancer dynamics. By disseminating this knowledge, health professionals can empower individuals to practice proactive skin care, fostering a culture of prevention that is vital for public health. This multifaceted approach to dermatological health is essential in addressing the complex interplay of factors that affect skin integrity and overall well-being.

Final Thoughts on Holistic Skin Wellness

In an era where the pursuit of skin health is often overshadowed by quick fixes and synthetic solutions, the importance of a holistic approach to skin wellness cannot be overstated. Integrating natural remedies, nutrition, and mindful practices into our daily routines offers a comprehensive path to achieving and maintaining skin vitality. This approach not only addresses existing skin conditions but also promotes overall wellness, recognizing the interconnectedness of body, mind, and environment. For health professionals guiding patients toward optimal skin health, understanding and advocating for holistic strategies is essential.

Natural remedies have been employed across cultures for centuries, providing effective solutions for various skin issues. Herbal treatments, for example, often offer anti-inflammatory and antioxidant properties that can enhance skin health while minimizing side effects commonly associated with pharmaceutical interventions. It is crucial for health professionals to evaluate these remedies scientifically, ensuring they can recommend safe and effective options to patients dealing with conditions such as eczema, psoriasis, or acne. By fostering a dialogue around these treatments, professionals can empower individuals to take an active role in their skin care.

Post-tattoo skin health is another critical aspect of holistic wellness that deserves attention. The skin's integrity must be preserved during the healing process, and guidelines for tattoo aftercare play a significant role in preventing complications. Educating clients about proper aftercare, including the use of barrier creams and natural moisturizers, can enhance healing and reduce the risk of infections. Such practices not only safeguard the skin but also promote a deeper understanding of its needs, reinforcing the importance of nurturing skin health through informed choices.

The role of nutrition in skin health cannot be overlooked. A well-balanced diet rich in vitamins, minerals, and antioxidants significantly influences skin conditions and the aging process. Health professionals should encourage individuals to consider how their dietary choices impact their skin, reinforcing the notion that true beauty is cultivated from within. By providing guidance on nutritional strategies tailored to specific skin types and conditions, practitioners can help clients achieve more radiant and resilient skin while addressing underlying health concerns.

Finally, fostering awareness around skin cancer prevention and management is paramount. Education on risk factors, protective measures, and the signs of skin cancer empowers individuals to take proactive steps in safeguarding their skin. This awareness, coupled with a holistic understanding of skin health, creates a comprehensive framework for maintaining skin integrity. As we conclude our exploration of holistic skin wellness, it is evident that a multifaceted approach, integrating natural remedies, nutrition, and preventive care, is essential for achieving not only healthier skin but also improved overall well-being.

www.ingramcontent.com/pod-product-compliance
Lightning Source LLC
Chambersburg PA
CBHW050319230526
45471CB00005B/2267